The
Essential
Nutrients

Adopting Healthy Habits

By

Dr.Michael F. Guion

Table of contents

Most of the time, we all want more energy, especially when we think about losing weight. When we alter our food intake patterns or reduce our overall caloric intake, it is common to experience a lack of energy. At these times, it's a higher priority than

ever for our food to give us that additional jolt of energy.

This is one justification for why nutrient-rich World's Best Food sources are so

beneficially assist you with feeling stimulated while shedding pounds.

And the process is quite straightforward: By providing your body with sufficient quantities of the nutrients required by the body's energy production systems, the World's Healthiest Foods can energize you.

It's not just that they give you enough of the macronutrients (carbohydrates, protein, and fat) that start the process of making energy. They additionally contain micronutrients (nutrients

what're more, minerals) that assistance to deliver the energy and afterward recover it so it tends to be put away for later use when and where it's generally required.

Your cells are where you get energy from your food. Probably the main energy creation spots are very little microstructures inside our phones called mitochondria. The process by which our mitochondria generate energy is difficult to comprehend. It depends on several enzymes that need a lot of important nutrients to work properly, like vitamins B1, B2, B3, B5, and B6, lipoic acid, coenzyme Q, iron, magnesium, and sulfur. In this way, envision the distinction in how much energy you'll feel from eating supplement poor refined food varieties rather than nutrient-rich entire food varieties like new natural products, mixed greens, and vegetables. In addition to these and other World's Healthiest Foods, they will unquestionably ensure that your energy systems receive the health-promoting nutrients they require to sustain your vitality.

Additionally, phytonutrients, which serve as potent antioxidants, can be found in the World's Healthiest Foods, particularly in fruits and vegetables. These nutrients derived from plants are capable of supporting healthy energy production in addition to the numerous other advantages they provide. This is because as your body generates energy, it also produces oxygen radicals that have the potential to harm the energy centers in the mitochondria as well as numerous cells and tissues, resulting in decreased and inefficient energy production. However, the nutrient-dense World's Healthiest Foods' phytonutrients and other antioxidants, such as vitamin E, can protect your cells by neutralizing oxygen radicals and preventing their damage.

Chapter.1

Changing Your Eating Routine: Picking Supplement rich Food varieties.

Pick an eating routine made of supplement-rich food varieties. Supplement-rich (or supplement-thick) food varieties are low in sugar, sodium, starches, and awful fats. They contain a lot of nutrients and minerals and scarcely any calories. Your body needs nutrients and minerals, known as micronutrients. They sustain your body and assist with keeping you solid. They can lessen your gamble for ongoing infections. Helping them through food guarantees your body can ingest them appropriately.

Attempt to eat various food sources to get various nutrients and minerals. Food sources that normally are supplement rich incorporate products of the soil. Lean meats, fish, entire grains, dairy, vegetables, nuts, and seeds additionally are high in supplements.

Way to further developed well-being.

You may not get every one of the micronutrients your body needs. Americans will generally eat food varieties that are high in calories and low in micronutrients. These food sources frequently additionally contain added sugar, sodium (salt), and immersed or trans fats. This sort of diet adds to weight gain. It can expand your gamble of medical problems, like sort 2 diabetes and coronary illness.

As indicated by the U.S. Branch of Horticulture (USDA), American grown-ups may not get enough of the accompanying micronutrients.

Supplement,

Food sources.

Calcium.

Nonfat and low-fat dairy, dairy substitutes, broccoli, dim, salad greens, and sardines

Potassium.

Bananas, melon, raisins, nuts, fish, spinach, and other dim greens

Fiber.
Vegetables (dried beans and peas), entire grain food sources and wheat, seeds, apples, strawberries, carrots, raspberries, and vivid products of the soil

Magnesium.

Spinach, dark beans, peas, and almonds

Vitamin A.
Eggs, milk, carrots, yams, and melon

L-ascorbic acid.
Oranges, strawberries, tomatoes, kiwi, broccoli, and red and green chile peppers

Vitamin E.
Avocados, nuts, seeds, entire grain food sources, and spinach and other dim mixed greens
The above food sources are all great decisions. The following are ideas for changing your eating regimen to be more supplement rich.

Grains.

Entire grain food sources are low in fat. They're additionally high in fiber and complex carbs. This assists you with feeling full longer and forestalls indulging. Check the fixing list for "entire." For instance, "entire wheat flour" or "entire oat flour." Search for items that have no less than 3 grams of fiber for each serving. A few improved flours have fiber yet are not supplement rich.

Pick these food sources:

- Rolled or steel-cut oats
- Entire wheat pasta
- Entire wheat tortillas
- Entire grain (wheat or rye) wafers, pieces of bread, and rolls
- Brown or wild rice
- Grain, quinoa, buckwheat, entire corn, and broken wheat

Foods grew from the ground.

Foods grown from the ground normally are low in fat. They add supplements, flavor, and assortment to your eating regimen. Search for bright leafy foods, particularly orange and dull green.

Pick these food sources:

- Broccoli, cauliflower, and Brussels sprouts
- Mixed greens, like chard, cabbage, romaine, and bok choy
- Dull, mixed greens, like spinach and kale
- Squash, carrots, yams, turnips, and pumpkin

- Snap peas, green beans, ringer peppers, and asparagus
- Apples, plums, mangos, papaya, pineapple, and bananas
- Blueberries, strawberries, cherries, pomegranates, and grapes
- Citrus organic products, like grapefruits and oranges
- Peaches, pears, and melons
- Tomatoes and avocados

Meat, poultry, fish, and beans.

Meat, pork, veal, and sheep.
Pick low-fat, lean cuts of meat. Search for the words "round," "midsection," or "leg" in their names. Cut back external excess before cooking. Trim any inside, detachable fat before eating. Baking, searing, and broiling are the best ways of setting up these meats. Limit how frequently you eat meat, pork, veal, and sheep. Indeed, even lean cuts contain more fat and cholesterol contrasted with other protein sources.

Poultry.

Chicken bosoms are a decent cut of poultry. They are low in fat and high in protein. Eliminate skin and outside fat before cooking. Baking, cooking, barbecuing, and broiling are the best ways of getting ready poultry.

Fish.

New fish and shellfish ought to be clammy and clear in variety. They ought to smell clean and have firm, springy tissue. If new fish isn't accessible, pick frozen or low-salt canned fish. Wild-got sleek fish are the best wellsprings of omega-3 unsaturated fats. This incorporates salmon, fish, mackerel, and sardines. Poaching, steaming, baking, and searing are the best ways of getting ready to fish.

Beans and other non-meat sources.

Non-meat wellsprings of protein additionally can be supplement rich. Attempt a serving of beans, peanut butter, different nuts, or seeds.

Pick these food varieties.

- Lean cuts of hamburger, pork, veal, and sheep
- Turkey bacon
- Ground chicken or turkey
- Wild-caught salmon and other slick fish
- Haddock and other white fish

- Wild-caught fish (canned or new)
- Shrimp, mussels, scallops, and lobster (without added fat)
- Vegetables, like beans, lentils, and chickpeas
- Seeds and nuts, including nut margarine

Dairy and dairy substitutes.

Pick skim milk, low-fat milk, or enhanced milk substitutes. Take a stab at supplanting cream with vanished skim milk in recipes and espresso. Pick low-fat or without-fat cheeses.

Pick these food sources.

- Low-fat, skim, nut, or advanced milk, similar to soy or rice
- Skim ricotta cheddar instead of cream cheddar
- Low-fat curds
- String cheddar
- Plain nonfat yogurt instead of acrid cream

Interesting points.

Most supplement-rich food sources are tracked down at the edge (external circle) of the supermarket. How much supplement-rich food varieties you ought to eat relies upon your everyday calorie needs. USDA's site ChooseMyPlate.gov offers sustenance data for grown-ups and kids.

Inquiries to pose to your primary care physician.

- How might I effectively add these food varieties to my ordinary eating routine?
- How might I be certain I'm eating an adequate number of supplement-rich food sources in the event that I'm on a severe eating routine, similar to a veggie lover or vegetarian?
- Could I at any point take enhancements or multivitamins to expand my supplements?

Chapter.2

Food.

Food is fundamental for everybody, assuming a part in our lives from customary days to extraordinary events and occasions. Gain proficiency with the significance of every nutritional category and how to design and plan nutritious feasts and snacks in a protected manner appropriately.

Wellbeing.

Dietary necessities change through each phase of life. A fair eating plan that spotlights nutritious food varieties and refreshments can assist with guaranteeing you're getting an adequate number of fundamental supplements to keep up with ideal wellbeing or oversee medical issues.

Fundamental Supplements.

Find out about micronutrients like nutrients and minerals, as well as macronutrients including protein, sugars, and fat. Get data on when enhancements might be justified, in addition to perceiving how much water you want to remain sufficiently hydrated.

Sugars.

Energizing wellsprings of sugars give supplements to assist with powering the body and advance great well-being.

Kids Need Sugars.

As of late, a few prevailing fashion counts calories have suggested the decrease, or even disposal, of carbs from our everyday eating schedule. However, are these "low carb" eats less great for youngsters? While decreasing particular sorts of carbs, like those with added sugars, is helpful, it isn't to eliminate all carbs.

Best Sugar Decisions.

The favored fuel for dynamic minds and developing muscles, sugars are tracked down in various food varieties. Milk and yogurt, pears and berries, potatoes and beans, rice and grain — all contain starches. As do improved drinks like pop, cakes, treats, and candy.

The best carb decisions give various supplements to assist with filling developing bodies and advance great well-being: nutrients, minerals, and dietary fiber. Instances of supplement-rich starches incorporate entire grains, vegetables, organic products, lentils, peas, and beans.

Low-endlessly fat-free milk and yogurt are other supplements rich in starch that gives calcium, and potassium and is invigorated with vitamin D.

Food varieties and beverages with added sugars are better saved as an intermittent treat since they don't offer nourishment past a fast energy source. These "periodic treats" incorporate soft drinks and other improved drinks, sweets, cakes, and treats.

The 2020-2025 Dietary Rules for Americans prescribe restricting added sugars to something like 10% of all calories each day beginning at age 2. Wellsprings of added sugars ought to be kept away from youngsters younger than 2. Check the Nourishment Realities Mark for how much-added sugars per serving.

Arriving at Everyday Dietary Fiber Needs.

White bread, pasta, and white rice are wellsprings of starches. Notwithstanding, they are refined and low in dietary fiber. Making half of your grains entire grains is a better direction for living for yourself as well as your loved ones. There are numerous delectable entire-grain choices including saltines, bread, pasta, cereals, freekeh, bulgur, earthy-colored rice, and entire-grain corn tortillas. Different models incorporate entire wheat roti, chapati, buckwheat, millet, and grain.

Alternate ways of remembering more dietary fiber for your kid's day incorporate picking entire organic products rather than 100 percent organic product squeeze and including vegetables.

Kids have different dietary fiber needs relying on their age:

- Youngsters 1 to 3 years: 19 grams of fiber each day
- Youngsters 4 to 8 years: 25 grams of fiber each day
- Females 9 to 18 years: 26 grams of fiber each day
- Guys 9 to 13 years: 31 grams of fiber each day
- Guys 14 to 18 years: 38 grams of fiber each day

Check the Nourishment Realities Name for how much dietary fiber per serving. A decent wellspring of dietary fiber has something like 3 grams of fiber for each serving; a phenomenal wellspring of dietary fiber has no less than 6 grams for every serving.

Going Gluten Free?;.

Sans gluten eating isn't the objective for everybody, except for youngsters with celiac infection or non-celiac gluten responsiveness, all wellsprings of gluten should be kept away from. Gluten is a protein, however, it's tracked down in specific grains, like wheat, rye, grain, and oats that are not handled in a sans-gluten office. Gluten items are accessible in numerous supermarkets and eateries, making it more straightforward for people who should conform to sans-gluten eating.

Certain individuals cut out gluten for a similar explanation they cut out carbs, however except if your youngster has been determined to have a condition like celiac sickness or non-celiac gluten responsiveness, it isn't required.

Chapter.3

Starches — Some portion of an Invigorating Diabetes Diet.

A typical nourishment legend is that people with diabetes need to keep away from starches. While people with diabetes should be aware of the number of sugars they eat, they don't have to keep away from them through and through. Carbs are the body's favored wellspring of fuel and food sources containing carbs can offer various nutrients, minerals, and different supplements.

There are three sorts of carbs: starches, sugars, and dietary fiber.

- Starches are available in plant-based food sources like potatoes, peas, corn, beans, rice, and other grain items.
- Sugars happen normally in food sources like products of the soil, yet there are additional wellsprings of added sugars that are tracked down in profoundly handled food sources, like sweets, cake, and soda pops.
- Dietary Fiber is a toxic piece of plant food sources that might assist with stomach-related and heart well-being.

People with diabetes ought to zero in on picking carbs from supplement-rich, entire food varieties like organic products, vegetables, beans, entire grains, and dairy items, including low-fat or sans-fat milk and yogurt. Food varieties and drinks with added sugars ought to be drunk sparingly, no matter what a diabetes conclusion.

Spreading carb decisions uniformly for the day assists with forestalling spikes and plunges in glucose. An enlisted dietitian nutritionist can make a particular dinner plan that fits individual inclinations with the exceptional necessities of somebody with diabetes.

Proposals for carb objectives will shift from one individual to another. For somebody who eats 2,000 calories every day, an RDN might suggest that one dinner contains around 45 to 60 grams of starch — or three to four servings of carbs. This might shift relying on how regularly an individual intends to eat over the course of the day.

In feast anticipating diabetes, a serving of sugars is equivalent to 15 grams of starch. Here are a few instances of serving sizes, however, allude to the Nourishment Realities Mark at whatever point workable for definite sums:

- New, frozen, or canned natural product:

1 little apple, a 4-inch long extra-little banana, or a medium orange

½ cup natural product mixed drink, canned pineapple or unsweetened fruit purée

- Dried organic product:

2 tablespoons of raisins or dried cranberries

- Endlessly milk Substitutes:

1 cup (8 liquid ounces) without fat, low-fat, or sans lactose milk

1 cup (8 liquid ounces) of unsweetened or light soy refreshments

- Yogurt:

⅔ cup (6 ounces) unsweetened or light assortments

- Cereal:

½ cup cooked cereal or cornmeal

½ cup grain pieces or plain destroyed wheat

- Entire grains:

⅓ cup cooked earthy-colored rice, quinoa, or entire wheat pasta

- Different starches:

½ burger bun or English biscuit

1 little (6-inch) corn or flour tortilla

- Bland vegetables:

½ cup crushed or bubbled potatoes

½ cup green peas or corn

½ cup dark, kidney, pinto, or garbanzo beans

- Desserts and different sugars:

1 tablespoon standard syrup, jam, jam, sugar or honey

½ cup sans sugar pudding

½ cup frozen yogurt

For the two individuals with and without diabetes, sugars assume a significant part in an energizing eating regimen.

Entire food varieties, for example, products of the soil, beans, entire grains, nuts, and seeds give dietary fiber, protein, and supplements to help well-being. Meet with an enrolled dietitian nutritionist to foster

an individualized dinner plan that works for you.

Chapter.4

Simple Methods for Helping Fiber in Your Day-to-Day Diet.

Fiber is a fundamental supplement. Notwithstanding, numerous Americans miss the mark concerning the suggested everyday sum in their weight control plans. Ladies ought to hold back nothing grams of fiber each day, while men ought to focus on around 38 grams or 14 grams for every 1,000 calories.

Dietary fiber adds to well-being and health in various ways. In the first place, it supports giving totality after dinners, which advances a solid weight. Second, satisfactory fiber admission can assist with bringing down cholesterol. Third, it prevents clogging and diverticulosis. What's more, fourth, sufficient fiber from food assists with blood sugar levels inside a sound reach.

Regular Wellsprings of Fiber.

Fiber is tracked down in plant food varieties. Eating the skin or strip of products of the soil gives a more noteworthy portion of fiber, which is tracked down normally in these sources. Fiber likewise is tracked down in beans and lentils, entire grains, nuts, and seeds. Commonly, the more refined or handled food is, the lower its fiber content. For instance, one medium apple with the strip holds back 4.4 grams of fiber, while ½ cup of fruit purée contains 1.4 grams, and 4 ounces of the squeezed apple contains no fiber.

By including specific food varieties, you can build your fiber admission in a matter of seconds. For breakfast, pick steel-cut oats with nuts and berries rather than a low-fiber, refined oat. At lunch, have a sandwich or wrap on an entire grain tortilla or entire grain bread and add veggies, like lettuce and tomato, or present with veggie soup. For a tidbit, have new veggies or entire grain wafers with hummus. With supper, attempt earthy-colored rice or entire-grain noodles rather than white rice or pasta made with white flour.

The following are a couple of food varieties that are normally high in fiber.

- 1 enormous pear with skin (7 grams)
- 1 cup new raspberries (8 grams)
- ½ medium avocado (5 grams)
- 1-ounce almonds (3.5 grams)
- ½ cup cooked dark beans (7.5 grams)
- 3 cups air-popped popcorn (3.6 grams)
- 1 cup cooked pearled grain (6 grams)

While expanding fiber, make certain to do it steadily and with a lot of liquids. As dietary fiber goes through the intestinal system, it is like another wipe; it needs water to fill up and pass without a hitch. Assuming you consume more than your standard admission of fiber yet insufficient liquid, you might encounter queasiness or blockage.

Before you go after the fiber supplements, think about this: fiber is tracked down normally in nutritious food sources. Studies have tracked down similar advantages, like a sensation of totality, that may not result from fiber supplements or fiber-improved food sources. On the off chance that you're passing up your day-to-day measure of fiber, you might be following in other fundamental supplements too. Your fiber admission is a decent measure for by and large eating routine quality. Attempt to arrive at your fiber objective with crude food varieties so you get the wide range of various advantages they give also.

Starches Fiber.

Natural products, vegetables, beans, and entire grains all contain dietary fiber, a kind of carb that gives negligible energy to the body. Albeit the body can't utilize fiber proficiently for fuel, it's a significant piece of a good dieting plan and assists with an assortment of medical issues.

Coronary illness: Fiber might assist with forestalling coronary illness by decreasing cholesterol.

Weight the board: Fiber eases back the speed at which food passes from the stomach to the remainder of the stomach-related framework - this can encourage us longer. Food varieties that are higher in dietary fiber frequently are lower in calories also.

Diabetes: Since fiber dials back how rapidly food is separated, it might assist with controlling glucose levels for individuals with diabetes by diminishing glucose levels after dinners.

Stomach-related issues: Fiber increments mass in the digestive system and may assist with working on the recurrence of solid discharges.

The suggested measure of dietary fiber is 14 grams for every 1,000 calories each day, or, around 25 grams for ladies and 38 grams for men every day. Your precise requirements might shift relying on your energy needs.

Entire grains and beans will generally be higher in fiber than foods grown from the ground, however, all are wellsprings of dietary fiber and offer other significant supplements. Make a point to incorporate different food varieties routinely to meet your dietary fiber needs. These are a couple of tips to assist with expanding your fiber consumption from food sources:

Blend in oats to meatloaf, bread, or other prepared products.
Prepare beans for your next salad or soup.
Hack up veggies to add to sandwiches or noodle dishes, for example, pasta or pan-fried food.
Mix natural products into a smoothie or use it to top oat, hotcakes, or sweets.
It likewise is vital to drink a lot of water and to build your fiber consumption progressively to give your body time to change.

Chapter.5

Fats.

Find out about the various sorts of dietary fats, some of which are more fortifying to eat than others. In late years, omega-3 unsaturated fats have become something of a sustenance star. In any case, what are they?

Omega-3s are fundamental unsaturated fats that assist with taking care of the mind and keeping it solid. They are important for the method involved with building new cells — the way to foster the focal apprehensive and cardiovascular frameworks and assist the body with retaining supplements. Omega-3 fats likewise are significant for eye capability.

Furthermore, some examination has shown omega-3 fats might assist with overseeing mental and social circumstances on account of their part in synapse capability. Concentrations on Japanese kids have demonstrated fish admission to be contrarily connected with burdensome side effects. Furthermore, the calming impacts of omega-3 fats have likewise been concentrated as an expected treatment for conditions going from weight to asthma to upper respiratory diseases.

Remember that a portion of these investigations were little and different examinations tracked down clashing outcomes. Additionally, the examination might have zeroed in on just a single kind of omega-3 unsaturated fat. More examination should be finished before we will know the full ramifications of omega-3 fats on the body. Continuously talk with your kid's medical care supplier before giving them any dietary enhancements.

3 Sorts of Omega-3 Fats.

The sorts of omega-3 fats are
- eicosapentaenoic corrosive (EPA),
- docosahexaenoic corrosive (DHA)
- , and alpha-linolenic corrosive (ALA).

EPA and DHA are tracked down fundamentally in specific fish, albeit certain brands of eggs might be braced. ALA is found basically in plant sources including flaxseed, chia seeds, and pecans, in addition to some fish and meat. Grass-treated creatures will generally have a higher measure of omega-3 unsaturated fats and produce milk and eggs with more too.

Food Before Enhancements.

Offer an assortment of food wellsprings of omega-3 fats before attempting supplements. Serve fish in kid-accommodating ways, for example, baking salmon in teriyaki or honey grill sauce. Utilize canned salmon to make salmon sliders, salmon cakes, or heated pieces. Servings of fish are more modest for youngsters and will rely upon their age. It's likewise essential to pick fish that are lower in mercury, for example, the ones recorded underneath. More "Counsel about Eating Fish" can be found on the U.S. Food and Medication Organization's site.

On the off chance that your children aren't into fish, take a stab at utilizing flaxseed oil. You can add a teaspoon to a smoothie or stir it up with peanut butter for toast and sandwiches. You can likewise add ground flax seeds to biscuits, soups, and even breadcrumbs before baking meals or chicken cutlets. Make pudding utilizing chia seeds and add your child's number one natural product for a supplement-pressed breakfast or tidbit.

The ongoing Suggested Sufficient Admissions of omega-3s for youngsters are:

- 0 to a year: 0.5 grams/day
- 1 to 3 years: 0.7 grams/day
- 4 to 8 years: 0.9 grams/day
- 9 to 13 years (young men): 1.2 grams/day
- 9 to 13 years (young ladies): 1.0 grams/day
- 14 to 18 years (young men): 1.6 grams/day

- 14 to 18 years (young ladies): 1.1 grams/day

To meet the everyday requirements of omega-3 fats for youngsters, search for these food sources:

- Salmon
- Sardines
- Pacific Chub Mackerel
- Canned light fish
- Freshwater Trout
- Herring
- Shellfish
- Shrimp
- Meat
- Flaxseeds
- Pecans
- Chia seeds
- Soybeans

Cerebrum Well-Being and Fish.

When was the last time you had fish for supper? On the off chance that you can't recollect, it could be more than the progression of time that is at fault. The research proposes that superior memory is only one of many mind-helping benefits related to eating more fish.

For getting healthy, the kind of food you eat is everything.

You've probably heard that omega-3 unsaturated fats are great for your well-being. However, one specifically, docosahexaenoic corrosive, or DHA, goes directly to your head. DHA is an omega-3 unsaturated fat that is expected to keep the mind working regularly and productively. Cerebrum and sensory system tissues are halfway composed of fat, and examination proposes they have an extraordinary inclination for DHA over different sorts of unsaturated fats.

Assuming you figure more significant levels of DHA in your eating regimen could assist you with making sure to put fish on your shopping list, remember that few examinations have connected DHA lacks to additional serious mental issues than periodic neglect. Truth be told, low degrees of DHA have been related to a more serious gamble of Alzheimer's sickness in later years.

Indications of cognitive decline ought not to be your most memorable sign to help admission. Consider fish utilization an investment funds plan for your mind, not a triumphant lottery ticket. Long-haul utilization of satisfactory DHA is connected to further developed memory and diminished paces of mental deterioration. To receive the mind rewards of DHA, you want to keep a reliable admission of DHA-rich food varieties.

Chapter.6

Ocean Commendable Servings.

Do you need to be swimming in fish suppers to take care of your cerebrum? The 2020-2025 Dietary Rules for Americans suggests grown-ups devour something like 8 ounces of fish each week. This works out to be two 4-ounce servings of fish. Sleek fish, for example, salmon, fish, Atlantic mackerel, herring, and trout are incredible with DHA to offer. At the point when you get cooking, think searing or barbecuing — the additional fat from profound broiling is counterproductive when there's rest protein on the menu. Pick assortments that are lower in mercury levels on a more regular basis, similar to salmon or freshwater trout. In the meantime, sharks and swordfish are being restricted because of high mercury levels. You likewise can choose fish that have a lesser natural effect - consider assortments that have been confirmed for capable fish creation.

Minds and Muscle.

Add another in addition to the fish list: lean protein. To ensure the body stays in top high-impact condition to muscle through the workout, the impact of fish on the heart is only another advantage. Besides being lower in soaked fat than red meat, trading burgers for fish implies more omega-3s, which studies recommend may diminish the gamble for coronary illness.

Fish or Ocean Growth?

For people who follow veggie lovers or vegetarians abstain from food, everything's not lost — it is possible to get DHA. Green growth is an essential wellspring of DHA and is utilized to make vegan DHA supplements. Ground flax seed, pecans, and chia seeds are other plant-based wellsprings of another omega-3 unsaturated fat, ALA, which the body changes over into DHA. In any case, our bodies might change over 15% of ALA to DHA. If your essential admission of omega-3s comes from sources other than slick fish, think about addressing a specialist or enrolled dietitian nutritionist regarding supplementation.

What are Omega-3 Unsaturated fats?

Research shows that eating two 4-ounce servings of fish each week might diminish the gamble of coronary illness and related passings. Numerous well-being experts trait this possibly life-saving nature of fish to the presence of omega-3 fundamental unsaturated fats. Furthermore, omega-3s are not restricted to fish and fish. They are likewise tracked down in a few vegetable oils, nuts, seeds, and soy food varieties.

Fish contain two significant omega-3 unsaturated fats: EPA (eicosapentaenoic corrosive) and DHA (docosahexaenoic corrosive). The research proposes individuals who eat greasy fish and other fish as a feature of a solid dietary example has the lower hazard of heart issues and lower dangers of constant illness. This has been found in people with and without a background marked by coronary illness, however, the proof is more grounded in the advantages of omega-3 unsaturated fats in individuals with a background marked by coronary illness. For example, assuming you have high blood fatty oils, consuming omega-3 unsaturated fats might assist with bringing down your levels.

Plant-Based Omega-3s.

A few plants likewise contain an omega-3 unsaturated fat known as ALA (alpha-linolenic corrosive). You can track it in different oils, nuts, seeds, beans, and different sources. Here are ways to get more plant-based omega-3s:

Incorporate oils that contain omega-3 unsaturated fats, for example, flaxseed oil, pecan oil, canola oil, or soybean oil.

Add hemp hearts or ground flaxseed to oats, yogurt, and mixed greens. The body can't separate entire flax seeds yet crushing them before use assists with ingestion.

Substitute ground flaxseed for part of the spread or oil while baking. Utilize 3 tablespoons of ground flaxseed blended in with 1 tablespoon of water to supplant 1 tablespoon of oil.

Nibble on edamame or pecans for a bite that gives omega-3 unsaturated fats.

Omega-3 Enhancements.

Omega-3 enhancements might be valuable in battling coronary illness however late examinations have tested on the off chance that taking enhancements is as successful as devouring food sources. Logical proof depicting the benefit of omega-3 enhancements on coronary illness risk for individuals who don't have a coronary illness is likewise restricted. Counsel a well-being expert to decide whether you would profit from an omega-3 enhancement.

An excessive amount of Omega-3?

Provided the reality that large numbers of our food varieties are braced with omega-3 unsaturated fats, it is possible to get abundance measures of it assuming you take extra enhancements. The U.S. Food and Medication Organization prompts eating something like 3 grams of EPA and DHA omega-3 unsaturated fats each day from food sources and dietary enhancements, except if recommended by a medical care supplier. Taking an excessive amount may cause awkward gastrointestinal side effects. Furthermore, albeit little, there is a gamble of expanded draining conceivable when individuals who take hostile to platelet specialists or anticoagulants likewise take high portions of omega-3 unsaturated fats.

The omega-3 unsaturated fat substance of fish differs. Higher sums are normally found from sources like herring, salmon, sardines, and trout. Mackerel is likewise a rich wellspring of omega-3 unsaturated fats, notwithstanding, one assortment known as ruler mackerel is likewise high in mercury, and the FDA prompts

Chapter.7

What is Cholesterol?

Cholesterol is a waxy substance found in creature-based food varieties that we eat and in our body's cells. Our bodies need cholesterol to work ordinarily and can make all the cholesterol it needs. Cholesterol in the body is utilized to make chemicals and vitamin D. It likewise assumes a part in the processing.

There are three principal sorts of cholesterol in the body:

- High-thickness lipoprotein, or HDL. Frequently called the great cholesterol, HDL assists with eliminating the overabundance of cholesterol from your body.

- Low-thickness lipoprotein, or LDL. LDL is the terrible or "crummy" cholesterol. It can prompt the development of plaque in the courses.
- Exceptionally low-thickness lipoprotein, or VLDL. VLDL likewise will in general advance plaque development.

One more substance remembered for lipid lab tests is fatty oil levels. Fatty substances are a particular sort of fat in the blood. High fatty substances might be an indication that you have overabundant muscle versus fat or might be at an expanded gamble for Type 2 diabetes. They likewise might be a sign that you are eating such a large number of calories, particularly from refined grains or food sources and drinks with added sugars. Fatty substances likewise can be raised in individuals who smoke or drink an excess of liquor.

Assuming that there is an excessive amount of cholesterol in the body, it develops. The waxy development, called plaque, adheres to the internal parts of the veins. As the conduits are limited and obstructed, it is challenging for the blood to move through them. The blockage can prompt blood coagulation, stroke, or coronary illness.

Am I In danger?

Numerous things might expand your gamble for elevated cholesterol, including:

- Hereditary qualities: Elevated cholesterol runs in certain families.
- Progress in years: As we age, our cholesterol levels rise.
- Meds: Certain medications can lift cholesterol levels.
- Corpulence: People with overweight or hefty weight records are at a more serious gamble for elevated cholesterol.
- Diet: Consuming high amounts of soaked and trans fats can raise LDL cholesterol levels.
- Inertia: Movement assists with raising HDL cholesterol.
- Smoking: Tobacco items decline HDL and increment LDL. The connection between smoking and elevated cholesterol is more prominent for ladies.

Elevated Cholesterol, What's going on?

Everybody with elevated cholesterol can profit from a heart-solid way of life. Notwithstanding, your PCP could prescribe extra help to deal with your cholesterol levels, similar to a cholesterol-bringing drug, particularly if your cholesterol is high as a direct result of hereditary qualities. Furthermore, assuming you are in danger of growing elevated cholesterol, basic way-of-life changes can assist with lessening that gamble. These incorporate eating a heart-solid eating regimen, being genuinely dynamic, and accomplishing or keeping a sound body weight.

With regards to a good dieting plan, four dietary changes might assist with holding your cholesterol in line:

Appreciate Food sources with Plant Sterols and Stanols.

A few food sources — organic products, vegetables, vegetable oils, nuts, seeds, and entire grains — contain substances called plant sterols and stanols. Eating food sources wealthy in these substances might assist with combating rising aggregate and LDL cholesterol levels. To expand your day-to-day consumption, likewise search for food varieties strengthened with plant sterols and stanols. For instance, some squeezed oranges, grains, and breakfast bars might be sustained.

fats are generally found in creature-based food sources like meats and entire-fat dairy items. Higher admissions of immersed fat have been found to raise LDL cholesterol. Studies have additionally demonstrated the way that supplanting wellsprings of soaked fat with unsaturated fats can assist with diminishing your aggregate and LDL cholesterol levels.

To assist with lessening your admission of immersed fat:

Cook with vegetable oils, like olive, canola, sunflower, and safflower.
Eat food sources wealthy in omega-3 unsaturated fats like salmon, pecans, and ground flaxseed.
Pick low-fat or without-fat dairy items, for example, 1% or skim milk and non-fat yogurt, or low-fat cheeses, for example, decreased-fat feta and part-skim mozzarella.
Trade out margarine and fat for vegetable oil choices, which offer unsaturated fats.
Stay away from trans fats — they have been found to expand LDL levels and were tracked down in profoundly handled food sources.

- Food makers have eliminated trans fats from their items, yet a few food varieties with a more drawn-out period of usability might in any case contain them. Check how much trans fat is on the Sustenance Realities Mark and in the fixings list. If it says the food contains a somewhat hydrogenated oil, set it back.

-

Select Lean Protein Food varieties.

Lean protein food varieties give fewer calories from fat. To pick lean cuts:

-
- Take a look at the bundle for the words flank or round.
- Take the skin off your chicken and turkey to diminish the soaked fat.
- Limit greasy, marbled meats, broiled or pan-fried food varieties, and different food sources that are high in soaked fat, like organ meats
- Pick better choices while eating out by choosing food varieties that are prepared, cooked, or barbecued.

Chapter.8

Appreciate Dissolvable Fiber.

Dietary fiber is tracked down in organic products, vegetables, beans, lentils, and entire grains. These supplement thick food sources give two sorts of fiber, solvent and insoluble. The two sorts are significant for good well-being. Getting sufficient measures of dietary fiber from various food varieties is significant for everybody.

Research has shown that dissolvable fiber, specifically, from natural products, vegetables, beans, lentils, and entire grains, may assist with bringing down LDL cholesterol. In the stomach, dissolvable fiber frames a thick, jam-like substance, which helps tie dietary cholesterol from the food varieties you're eating. Along these lines, load up on vegetables and organic products:

- Select foods are grown from the ground which additionally gives dissolvable fiber. For instance, figs, Brussels sprouts, peaches, carrots, apricots, mangoes, and oranges.
- Eat a wide range of hued leafy foods.
- Shift to more plant-based or vegan dinners by including beans, lentils, and soy food sources.
- Center around entire types of produce, which incorporates new, frozen, canned, or dried.

- Search for canned natural products stuffed in water or their juice.
- Pick low-sodium canned veggies or assortments with no added salt.

Entire grains likewise are an incredible method for getting the advantages of dietary fiber:

- Eat grain (not pearled) and oats — both of these give dissolvable fiber.
- Ensure the food name on your bread says 100 percent entire grain or records an entire grain as quite possibly the earliest fixing.
- Limit refined starches, particularly wellsprings of added sugars, for example, desserts and sugar-improved drinks.

One note of watchfulness: as you increment your fiber admission, likewise increment your admission of water. This will assist with diminishing your gamble of becoming obstructed. On the off chance that you find it hard to get sufficient dietary fiber every day through your food sources, ask your medical care supplier before considering a fiber supplement.

Fatty substances: What difference do they make?

Fatty substances are a sort of fat in the blood. Elevated degrees of fatty substances can expand your gamble for coronary illness. Fortunately, the very suggestions that are educated for a number regarding different circumstances —, for example, getting thinner, being truly dynamic, and restricting refined sugars — may likewise assist with bringing down fatty oils.

At the point when an excessive number of calories are eaten, the body stores them as fatty substances for use sometime in the not-too-distant future; however, when fatty oil levels become excessively high, they might increase the risk for coronary illness. An ordinary fatty substance level is viewed as under 150 mg/dL while a level over 200 mg/dL is high. For some, a solid level can be accomplished through the accompanying way of life changes.

An Emphasis on Fats.

Fat certainly stands out in heart-good dieting plans yet that doesn't mean you want to dispose of it. All things being equal, centers around supplanting wellsprings of soaked fat (like margarine) with unsaturated fats, like olive and vegetable oils, nuts and seeds, avocados, and greasy fish.

Notwithstanding different other advantageous supplements, many kinds of fish give omega-3 fundamental unsaturated fats which can assist with diminishing fatty substance levels. Counting an assortment of fish that are lower in mercury two times each week (around 8 ounces complete) is suggested for adults. Seafood higher in omega-3 unsaturated fats incorporates salmon, herring, Atlantic and Pacific mackerel, rainbow trout, and sardines. Note: People who are pregnant or nursing and have small kids ought to keep away from sharks, swordfish, lord mackerel, and tilefish, which contain elevated degrees of mercury. For more data, see Counsel about Eating Fish from the U.S. Food and Medication Organization and the U.S. Natural Security Office.

On the off chance that you have high or exceptionally high fatty substances, your primary care physician may likewise suggest a medicine portion of supplemental omega-3 unsaturated fats. This ought to just be finished under the counsel and management of a specialist.
Be Carb Sagacious
While additional calories from any source can be put away as fatty oils, overabundant calories from added sugars and liquor might affect raising fatty oils.

While picking starch-rich food varieties, center around entire grains, natural products, vegetables, and low-fat dairy. Limit refined grains and wellsprings of added sugars, for example, pastries, heated merchandise, and sugar-improved refreshments. Furthermore, limit or keep away from liquor

Mediterranean-style eating plans are also connected with further developed heart well-being. This incorporates eating more organic products, vegetables, entire grains, and fish while restricting immersed fat, added sugars, sodium, and liquor. It likewise incorporates a moderate measure of monounsaturated and polyunsaturated fats found in oils like canola and olive oils.

Counsel an Expert.

Assuming your fatty substance level is over 150 mg/dL, talk about your way of life changes with your primary care physician and enlisted dietitian nutritionist. An RDN can assist you with fostering a good dieting plan that meets your own well-being needs and way of life.

Chapter.9

Protein.

A fundamental macronutrient, protein is liable for building tissues in the body including muscle.

How Much Protein Should I Eat?.

Protein is a supplement tracked down in many sorts of food varieties. It is essential forever. Whenever your body is developing or fixing itself, protein is required. How much protein you want relies upon a few variables — including age, sex, well-being status, and movement level.

The body needs a customary stockpile of protein to make and fix cells. Notwithstanding muscles, other body tissues are produced using protein, similar to organs, hair, and eyes. This supplement additionally makes a difference:

- Battle contamination
- Convey fats, nutrients, minerals, and oxygen around the body
- Construct and agreement muscles
- Keep body liquids in balance
- Cluster blood

Food sources that Contain Protein.

Protein can be seen in both creature and plant-based food sources. A few wellsprings of protein are viewed as preferable decisions over others because of their impact on heart well-being. Eating plans that incorporate low-fat dairy items, skinless poultry, fish, beans, lentils and soy food varieties like tofu and tempeh may assist with further developing pulse and cholesterol levels.

Here are some nutritious protein food choices:

- Meat, poultry, and eggs: lean cuts of hamburger, sheep, goat, pork flank, skinless chicken and turkey, quail and duck
- Fish and fish: salmon, fish, cod, shrimp, mackerel, lobster, catfish, crab
- Low-fat or sans-fat dairy food varieties: yogurt, milk, cheddar, curds
- Vegetables: beans, split peas, lentils, soy

- Nuts and seeds: pecans, almonds, chia seeds, pumpkin seeds, pistachios, cashews, and peanuts

Food varieties wealthy in protein may likewise be high in immersed fat. High admissions of soaked fat might increase the risk of coronary illness. In this manner, an excess of protein from these sources might be unsafe for your heart. When in doubt, limit protein food sources that are high in immersed fats, for example,

- Meats and poultry: bacon, southern-style steak, Chorizo wiener, broiled chicken, franks, lunch meats, organ meats, handled meats, frankfurter, and extra ribs
- Fish and shellfish: breaded and broiled choices
- Entire-fat dairy: entire milk and other entire-fat dairy items

These proposals for protein are given in one-ounce reciprocals. One-ounce reciprocals of protein food varieties include:

- One ounce of cooked meat, poultry, or fish

- ¼ cup cooked beans
- 1 egg
- 1 tablespoon peanut butter
- ½ ounce nuts or seeds

Be that as it may, most normal servings of protein food varieties incorporate more than one ounce of protein. For instance, a piece of meat about the size of a deck of cards, a container of depleted fish, and a little chicken bosom half are around three ounce-counterparts of protein each. Moreover, entire grain and dairy food sources contain protein. Most Americans get sufficient protein by and large, yet moving their admission to incorporate fish two times every week and vegetables all the more frequently instead of other protein food varieties is empowered.

Protein Food Sources for Your Vegan Youngster.

Kids don't have to eat meat to get the essential protein to keep their bodies solid and developing. Vegan kids grow ordinarily and can address nourishing issues when their eating regimens are arranged suitably. Virtually all food varieties — including vegetables — contain a limited quantity of protein. Assemble dinners around these plant-based food sources that contain protein and are wealthy in supplements.

Tofu and Tempeh.

Tofu and tempeh pack protein and cell reinforcements. Furthermore, some are sustained with calcium. Utilize the surface of tofu as a manual to assist you with integrating it into dishes. Add smooth luxurious tofu to smoothies, soups, puddings, and plunges. Delicate tofu looks like ricotta cheddar or fried eggs and is best integrated into rice, pasta, or in sandwiches. Prepare pieces from extra-firm tofu or solid shape and sauté with pan sear vegetables. Tempeh is produced using matured soybeans, and its surface looks extra-firm and can be utilized along these lines. For additional flavor, marinate tofu and tempeh in a delightful sauce in the fridge a couple of hours before cooking.

Beans, Peas, and Lentils.

Beans, peas, and lentils offer protein, fiber, folate, potassium, and magnesium, and planning is straightforward. Lentils cook for 20 to 30 minutes while dousing dried beans for 4 hours, or short-term is suggested. Dispose of the splashing water and stew beans in new water for 60 to an hour and a half. On the other hand, you can concoct dried lentils and beans in a strain cooked to save time. Refrigerate cooked beans and use for something like four days or freeze them for a very long time. Canned beans and lentils are helpful, and if "no salt added" jars are inaccessible, channel and flush beans completely to eliminate close to a portion of the sodium.

Beans, peas, and lentils come in many sorts and varieties, making them amusing to analyze. Make a graph with your youngster and cook another assortment every week, and have them draw a smiley face close to their top choices. There are such countless kinds of beans, peas, and lentils to look over! A few assortments incorporate moong beans, dark-looking peas, red lentils or split red lentils, adzuki beans, kidney beans, dark beans, pinto beans, fava beans, chickpeas, cowpeas, and spread beans.

Add beans to soups, salsa, rice, and mixed greens. Make bean enchiladas or quesadillas or use refried beans to make burritos, tostadas or molletes. Add to barbecued cheddar sandwiches, scoop with corn chips, or puree into plunges or heated merchandise including treats or brownies. Use peas to make samosa; fava beans to make ful medames; soybeans to make natto; crushed peas to make Eskimo; and red beans to make red beans and rice. Cook chickpeas in the broiler for a crunchy nibble!

Nuts and Nut Spreads.

Guardians frequently ask what nuts are best, at the same time, as a general rule, they all are — giving protein, solid fats, selenium and vitamin E. Attempt crude unsalted nuts and regular nut spreads without salt, sugar, or to some degree hydrogenated vegetable oils. Joining nuts with food sources your youngster now eats likewise is a decent choice to get the advantages of nuts. Offer natural products for a reasonable tidbit, or load a small bunch with your youngster's number one saltines or dried natural product to go. Pistachios are amusing to a shell, while pecans, cashews, and pine nuts are delicate; almonds and walnuts are normally sweet. For breakfast, add slashed nuts to biscuits, bread, and flapjack hitters, or sprinkle on oats or low-sugar breakfast grain. Add to servings of mixed greens, rice, and quinoa. Nut margarine likewise tastes great when added to cereal and smoothies.

Building Muscle on a Veggie Lover Diet.

For a long time, the regular conviction that managed proficient and novice athletic preparation programs was that consuming meat was the best way to fabricate muscle. Today, we realize a fair vegan diet that incorporates plant-based protein helps a strong turn of events … no steak is required.

Very much arranged veggie lover slims down that address energy issues and contains an assortment of plant-based protein food sources, for example, soy items, beans, lentils, grains, nuts, and seeds can give satisfactory protein to competitors without the utilization of extraordinary food sources or enhancements. In any case, thoughts should be made for the kind of vegan diet a competitor follows:

- Veggie lover - a vegan diet that creates items, like meat, poultry, fish, eggs, milk, cheddar, and other dairy items, and which depends on plant protein just to address protein issues.
- Lactovegetarian - a veggie-lover diet that prohibits meat, poultry, fish, and eggs,

however, incorporates dairy items, similar to without fat or low-fat milk, yogurt, and cheddar, which are wellsprings of protein.

- Lacto-ovo veggie lover - a vegan diet that prohibits meat, poultry, and fish, however, incorporates eggs and dairy items, which are likewise wellsprings of protein.

Competitors need to eat a suitable measure of calories and an assortment of protein food varieties for the day to meet their protein prerequisites. Amino acids make up the protein that our bodies need. Meat, eggs, and dairy food sources are regularly the most sought-after protein sources since they contain every one of the nine fundamental amino acids in the proportions that people require. Most wellsprings of plant-based protein are deficient in no less than one of the nine fundamental amino acids. Soy and quinoa are two special cases. Counting an assortment of plant-based protein food sources will guarantee each of the fundamental amino acids is being devoured.

Eat Protein For the Day.

Veggie-lover competitors ought to incorporate a quality wellspring of protein with feasts and tidbits. Here are a few ways to address protein issues without consuming meat:

Eat five or six little dinners each day that incorporate a protein food, yet additionally different natural products, vegetables, entire grains, and a lot of water.

The greater part of your calories every day ought to come from quality starches, which fuel your muscles.

Pick heart-solid wellsprings of fat, similar to olive oil, almonds, pecans, avocados, and canola oil.

Find an enlisted dietitian nutritionist who can work with you to make a customized veggie-lover eating plan that meets your singular requirements.

Chapter.10

Vitamins.

Every one of the 13 vitamins plays an exceptional part to play in our general well-being.

Cancer prevention agents Safeguarding Sound Cells.

Our bodies are milestones against contamination and infections. Typical body capabilities, like breathing or actual work, and another way of life propensities (like smoking) produce substances called free revolutionaries that assault solid cells. At the point when these sound cells are debilitated, they are more vulnerable to cardiovascular sickness and specific sorts of diseases. Cell reinforcements —, for example, nutrients C and E and carotenoids, which incorporate beta-carotene, lycopene, and lutein —

assist with safeguarding sound cells from harm brought about by free revolutionaries.

Carotenoids.

Among the at least 600 carotenoids in food sources, beta-carotene, lycopene, and lutein are notable forerunners in the battle to diminish the harm from free extremists. Food sources high in carotenoids might be viable in forestalling specific tumors and may assist with diminishing your gamble of macular degeneration.

Food sources high in carotenoids incorporate red, orange, profound yellow, and a few dull green verdant vegetables; these incorporate yams, spinach, carrots, tomatoes, Brussels sprouts, winter squash, and broccoli.

Vitamin E.

Research plays showed the wide part of vitamin E in advancing well-being. The fundamental job of vitamin E is as a cell reinforcement. Research has taken a gander at its conceivable job in assisting with safeguarding your body from cell harm that can prompt malignant growth, coronary illness, and waterfalls as we age. Vitamin E works with different cancer prevention agents, for example, L-ascorbic acid to offer security from a few persistent infections. Vitamin E is tracked down in vegetable oils, raw grains, entire grains, braced cereals, seeds, nuts, and peanut butter.

L-ascorbic acid.(vitamin c)

Maybe the most popular cancer prevention agent, L-ascorbic acid offers a wide assortment of medical advantages. These advantages incorporate safeguarding your body from disease and harm to body cells, helping produce collagen (the connective tissue that keeps bones and muscles intact), and helping in the retention of iron.

To exploit these advantages, eat food varieties plentiful in L-ascorbic acid, for example, citrus organic products (counting oranges, grapefruits, and tangerines), strawberries, sweet peppers, tomatoes, broccoli, and potatoes.

Difficulties Stimulating Eating.

The most ideal way to construct a refreshing eating plan is to eat even feasts and snacks every day and to partake in a wide assortment of food sources. For most grown-ups, eating something like 1 1/2 cups of products of soil cups of vegetables every day is a decent beginning for invigorating living. Keep in mind: new, frozen, dried, and canned foods are grown from the ground are nutritious! Pick frozen and canned choices without added sugars or salt.

Numerous well-being specialists suggest getting cell reinforcements from food rather than enhancements, and examination has not demonstrated cancer prevention agent enhancements to be advantageous in forestalling sickness. Truth be told, now and again cell reinforcement supplements have expanded the gamble of specific tumors. In any case, there might be conditions that make energizing eating a test. Find out if you want an enhancement. An enrolled dietitian nutritionist can assess your eating design and decide if an enhancement is ideal for you.

What Is Vitamin D?

Vitamin D is a supplement required for well-being and to keep up areas of strength. Vitamin D guides in the retention of calcium and phosphorus in our bodies, carry calcium and phosphorus to our bones and teeth and manages how much calcium stays in our blood. Along with calcium, vitamin D safeguards against the deficiency of bone mass.

Vitamin D's significance doesn't end there. It likewise helps muscle capability and permits the mind and body to convey through nerves. The safe framework likewise utilizes vitamin D. There are three methods for getting vitamin D: from daylight, through food and beverages, or with supplements.

Vitamin D from the Sun.

Known as the "daylight nutrient," your body changes over daylight into vitamin D after it hits unprotected skin. In any case, be mindful to keep away from stretched-out openness to daylight without sunscreen.

Vitamin D from Food and Beverages.

Not many food varieties normally have vitamin D. Greasy fish, for example, salmon and trout are among the best wellsprings of vitamin D. Meat liver, cheddar and egg yolk give limited quantities. Mushrooms additionally contain this nutrient assuming developed under UV lights.

Strengthened food sources and beverages give the majority of the vitamin D in our weight control plans. Most milk and a few oats are invigorated with vitamin D, as are many plant-based refreshments, similar to soymilk. Squeezed orange, yogurt, and cheddar could be sustained, so it is in every case great practice to check the Sustenance Realities Mark for vitamin D substance.

Vitamin D from Enhancements.

A few people might require additional vitamin D, like more seasoned grown-ups; breastfed babies; individuals with brown complexion; those with specific ailments including liver sickness, cystic fibrosis, celiac illness, and Crohn's infection; and those with stoutness or who have had gastric detour a medical procedure. Continuously check with your medical care supplier before taking a vitamin D enhancement.

What Are B-Nutrients?

Eight notable B-nutrients assume a part of the body. They support digestion and add to the body's capacity to create energy. A few of the B-nutrients have extra capabilities too:

Vitamin B6:

On the other hand, known as pyridoxine, vitamin B6 assists with delivering insulin, battling contamination, and making unnecessary amino acids (the structure blocks of protein). Beans, chicken, bananas, potatoes, pork, fish, nuts, and sustained breakfast grains all contain vitamin B6.

Chapter.11

Folate.

Otherwise called a folic corrosive, folate is especially significant during pregnancy. Consuming sufficient sums assists with lessening the gamble of spine and mind deformations (known as brain tube absconds). Wellsprings of folate incorporate many products of the soil — including beans, oranges, avocado, and spinach. Folic corrosive is tracked down in enhanced grains, similar to bread and pasta, strengthened breakfast oats, and dietary enhancements.

Vitamin B12.

Cobalamin, or vitamin B12, assumes a significant part in making new red platelets and a lack could bring about weakness. It is available in creature items like meat, fish, poultry, eggs, and dairy food varieties, like milk, yogurt, and cheddar. Some morning meal grains are additionally braced with vitamin B12 and can be a significant wellspring of this nutrient for veggie lovers and vegetarians. Albeit, a vitamin B12 supplement may likewise be required.

These B-nutrients are more ordinarily known by their names than by their numbers, yet all are generally accessible in various food sources and lack is somewhat exceptional in the US:

- Thiamin: Pork, peas, entire grain, and improved grain items including bread, rice, pasta, tortillas, and invigorated oats.
- Riboflavin: Milk, cheddar, yogurt, improved grains, lean meats, eggs, almonds, and verdant green vegetables.
- Niacin: High-protein food sources like peanut butter, hamburger, poultry, and fish, as well as improved and invigorated grain items
- Pantothenic Corrosive: Yogurt, yams, milk, avocado, corn, eggs, and beans.

- Biotin: Eggs, peanuts, fish, yams, and almonds.

Lack of vitamin D in Children.

Made in the body from openness to daylight, vitamin D assumes a significant part in bone well-being alongside calcium. Vitamin D advances the assimilation of calcium and phosphorus and helps store these minerals in bones and teeth making them more grounded and better.

The fortress of cow's milk with vitamin D has enormously decreased the gamble of lack of vitamin D in youngsters. In any case, the rising utilization of juice and sodas instead of milk alongside less play time outside is expanding the gamble of lack among kids, which can prompt rickets or flawed bone development.

Youngsters more established than 1 year need 600 IU of vitamin D consistently. Ensure your kid is getting sufficient vitamin D by incorporating braced milk with feasts. For instance, one cup of sustained 1 percent milk contains around 100 IU. Fish, like salmon, mackerel, and fish, as well as egg yolks, and strengthened breakfast oats additionally contain vitamin D.

Chat with your kid's medical services supplier to decide whether your kid is meeting their vitamin D necessities or on the other hand if they might require an enhancement. For directions concerning serving fish to small kids, visit the U.S. Food and Medication Organization's site.

How Vitamin C Supports a Healthy Immune System.

L-ascorbic acid, or ascorbic corrosive, is a water-dissolvable nutrient notable for its part in supporting a sound-safe framework. Since your body can't make L-ascorbic acid, it should come from the food varieties you eat each day. Research shows that L-ascorbic acid is fundamental for the development and fixation of tissue all around the body. L-ascorbic acid mends wounds and fixes and keeps up with sound bones, teeth, skin, and ligament — a kind of firm tissue that covers the bones. As a cell reinforcement, L-ascorbic acid battles free extremists in the body which might help forestall or postpone specific tumors and coronary illness and advance solid maturing. L-ascorbic acid from food varieties additionally appears to diminish the gamble of ligament misfortune in those with osteoarthritis.

However it may not hold you back from getting a bug, there is some proof that high portions of L-ascorbic acid might diminish the length of cold side effects by as much as coordinated-and-a-half days for certain individuals. Nonetheless, different examinations didn't bring about similar discoveries, and the gamble of aftereffects is more prominent with high dosages of L-ascorbic acid enhancements, so check with your primary care physician or enrolled dietitian nutritionist before taking.

Wellsprings of L-ascorbic acid are bountiful and expand well past the consistently famous orange or squeezed orange. Many products of the soil supply this fundamental nutrient. Wellsprings of L-ascorbic acid incorporate citrus natural products, tomatoes, potatoes, strawberries, green and red ringer peppers, broccoli, Brussels sprouts, and kiwifruit, among others. You can partake in these food sources crude or cooked, yet it's essential to take note of the fact that products of the soil lose L-ascorbic acid when warmed or put away for significant periods. To get the most supplements, eat them quickly in the wake of shopping and think about steaming or microwaving vegetables for brief time frames to restrict supplement misfortune.

Vegans might be particularly intrigued to know that L-ascorbic acid assists the body with better retaining non-heme iron — the sort from plant food varieties like beans, spinach, and quinoa. To get this advantage, join L-ascorbic acid-rich food varieties with iron-rich plant food sources in a similar feast. For instance, consolidate dark beans and salsa or make a tasty spinach salad with strawberries and mandarin oranges.

Chapter.12

Minerals.

Minerals, like calcium and iron, are essential to keep our bodies working appropriately.

Calcium.

Calcium is maybe the most notable and fundamental supplement for bone well-being. Building solid bones resembles building a good overall arrangement in your "calcium financial balance." Bones are living tissue and continually in a condition of turnover, setting aside calcium installments and withdrawals day to day.

Bones don't accompany a lifetime. They need persistent upkeep or they can debilitate and break. Assuming your everyday intake of calcium is low, your body will take calcium from your issues that remain to be worked out, blood calcium at typical levels.

To fulfill calcium requirements and profit from a lifetime of strong bones:

- Polish off three servings of dairy or calcium-sustained soy renditions, for example, low-fat or sans-fat milk, soy milk, or yogurt, consistently.
- Pick verdant green vegetables, calcium-sustained tofu, canned sardines, and salmon with delicate bones for extra calcium sources.
- While choosing 100 percent organic product squeezes and prepared-to-eat oats, pick ones braced with calcium
- Be dynamic with weight-bearing exercises, for example, running, moving, or weight lifting

Focus on Food First .

Enlisted dietitian nutritionists (RDNs) suggest food as the essential wellspring of nutrients, minerals, and different supplements, like calcium.

While shopping read the Sustenance Realities Name and select food varieties that contain 10% or a greater amount of the Day to day Incentive for calcium. Food varieties that are normally high or invigorated with calcium might be marked as "calcium-rich" or "magnificent wellspring of calcium."

Searching for a speedy method for helping your calcium consumption? Attempt these simple tips:

- Drink an 8-ounce glass of low-fat milk or a calcium-braced refreshment, similar to soymilk, with your feasts. Sans fat and low-fat milk have a comparative measure of calcium as entire milk.
- Make oats with milk or a calcium-braced refreshment rather than water.
- Eat 1 cup of low-fat or sans-fat yogurt with natural products for breakfast or a tidbit.

- Top a heated potato with steamed broccoli and destroy low-fat or sans-fat cheddar. For extra calcium, substitute plain Greek yogurt for sharp cream.
- Add calcium-rich greens (like collard greens, turnip greens, or kale) to feasts.
- Appreciate ½ cup cooked soybeans or 5 dried figs for a tidbit.
- Make a morning meal shake by mixing milk or a calcium-invigorated refreshment with leafy foods green, similar to spinach.
- Appreciate calcium-sustained tofu as a plant-based protein choice. Other plant-based decisions that give protein and calcium incorporate soybeans, almond spread, and tempeh.

How Effectively Is Calcium Absorbable?.

Calcium is assimilated best on the off chance that your admission of calcium-rich food sources is fanned out during the day. An RDN can assist you with picking food sources or a mix of food sources and an enhancement to meet your singular calcium needs while remembering calcium admission shouldn't surpass 2,500 milligrams each day for grown-ups between ages 19 and 50. This sum is diminished to 2,000 milligrams each day for grown-ups more than 51.

More Tips for Bone Health.

While picking calcium-rich food varieties and taking part in weight-bearing exercises are critical to bone well-being, there are a couple of different tips to remember:

- Abstain from smoking and unreasonable liquor admission.
- Inquire as to whether you want a bone thickness test in light of your gamble factors for osteoporosis or on the other hand if you are a lady north of 50.
- If you want a calcium supplement, pick one that likewise contains vitamin D, which will support calcium retention.

If you don't know whether your dietary patterns are meeting your healthful requirements, think about seeing an RDN for individual direction and proposals.

Iodine: A Significant Supplement...

A fundamental mineral, iodine is utilized by the thyroid organ to make thyroid chemicals that control many capabilities in the body including development and improvement. Since your body doesn't deliver iodine, it should be provided in the eating routine. At the point when iodine admission is poor, the body can't deliver an adequate number of thyroid chemicals.

Iodine lack in pregnancy is an overall issue and has turned into a worldwide general well-being worry since it is recognized as the main source of preventable cerebrum harm in babies and newborn children because of deficient admission by moms and newborn children. Significant global endeavors are being made to assist with lessening the issue, primarily using iodized salt and enhancements.

Until the mid-1900s, iodine deficiency was a typical issue in the US however was essentially improved with the expansion of iodine to table salt. Hypothyroidism, thyroid organ expansion (goiter), and weight gain are different circumstances that might result from too little iodine in the eating regimen. Numerous pregnant ladies in the U.S. keep on having deficient iodine admissions, particularly the individuals who have low admissions of dairy, fish, and iodized salt.

Chapter.13

Iodine and the Cerebrum.

With iodine inadequacy recorded as the main source of scholarly inability all over the planet, iodine is a significant part of sound mental health. The most harmful outcomes are on fetal and newborn child improvement of the mind when lack can cause irreversible cerebrum harm that endures forever. Cerebrum harm, cretinism, scholarly incapacity, and different circumstances are extra dangers.

It is a vital supplement throughout life, particularly during pregnancy, earliest stages, and youth when thyroid chemicals control development in the creating cerebrum. Less serious iodine deficiency appears as less than ideal intelligence level in youngsters, remembering weakened mind capability for grown-ups as well. During adolescence, iodine lack is frequently connected with goiter and connected to diminished scholarly and engine execution, as well as an expanded gamble for ADHD in kids.

Iodine Prerequisites.

A teaspoon of iodine is everyone an individual expects in a lifetime, but since iodine can't be put away for significant stretches, limited quantities are required routinely. The Establishment of Medication, or IOM, suggested dietary remittances for iodine are:

- 1 to 8 years of age: 90 micrograms
- 9 to 13 years of age: 120 micrograms
- 14 years and more seasoned: 150 micrograms
- Pregnant: 220 micrograms
- Lactating: 290 micrograms

Best Sources of Iodine.

Iodine fortress is what most nations depend on to support satisfactory dietary admission. In the excess of 70 nations that iodized salt, it for the most part fills in as the significant wellspring of iodine consumption. One-fourth of a teaspoon of iodized salts has around 100 micrograms of iodine. Note that the salt utilized in handled food varieties, which is the significant wellspring of salt for most Americans, ordinarily doesn't contain iodine. On the off chance that salt utilized in a handled food contains iodine, it will be recorded in the fixings rundown of that food. Zero in on diminishing how much salt ate from handled food sources and get your sodium from iodized salt.

Ocean growth, saltwater fish, and fish are normal wellsprings of dietary iodine. Dairy items likewise supply iodine in the eating routine at different levels. During lactation, the bosom moves iodine in milk, so breastmilk tends to be a decent wellspring of iodine for however long the mother's iodine admission is sufficient.

Plants filled in iodine-rich soil are likewise great sources; in any case, this is not a solid wellspring of iodine since there is no chance of realizing whether produce bought in supermarkets is filled in iodine-rich soil.

Iodized salt generally adds not exactly around 300 micrograms of iodine day to day to the eating routine. Most multivitamin-mineral enhancements contain 150 micrograms of iodine. With the protected maximum constraint of day-to-day iodine consumption for grown-ups set at 1,100 micrograms by the IOM, it is probably not going to hit an overabundance sum while including a multivitamin and normal wellsprings of dietary iodine.

The pattern of eating less table salt, dairy, and bread has a few specialists worried that iodine lack could be on the ascent once more. Eating a sound, adjusted diet that incorporates iodine-rich food varieties and iodized salt is vital to great well-being. Pre-birth nutrients containing iodine can assist with addressing dietary requirements for pregnant and lactating moms.

Foods to Fight Iron Deficiency.

You might siphon iron at the exercise center a couple of times each week, yet your body siphons it through the circulation system consistently. Iron is expected to make hemoglobin, a piece of red platelets that behaves like a cab for oxygen and carbon dioxide. It gets oxygen in the lungs, drives it through the circulation system, and drops it off in tissues including the skin and muscles. Then, at that point, it gets carbon dioxide and drives it back to the lungs where it's breathed out.

Iron Deficiency.

If the body doesn't retain its required measure of iron, it becomes iron-lacking. Side effects show up just when lack of iron has advanced to press weakness, a condition in which the body's iron stores are low to such an extent that insufficient typical red platelets can be made to proficiently convey oxygen. Lack of iron is quite possibly the most well-known nourishing lack and the main source of pallor in the US.

Side effects include:

- Weakness
- Fair skin and fingernails
- Shortcoming
- Unsteadiness
- Migraine
- Glossitis (excited tongue)

Sources of Iron.

The body assimilates a few times more iron from creature sources than from plants. The absolute best creature wellsprings of iron are:

- Lean hamburger
- Shellfish
- Chicken
- Turkey

Even though you retain less of the iron in plants, each nibble counts, and adding a wellspring of L-ascorbic acid to vegan wellsprings of iron will upgrade retention. Probably the best plant wellsprings of iron are:

- Beans and lentils
- Tofu
- Prepared potatoes
- Cashews
- Dull green verdant vegetables like spinach
- Sustained breakfast grains
- Entire grain and improved bread

High-Risk Populations.

The accompanying populaces are at a higher gamble for creating a lack of iron.

Ladies Who Are Pregnant: Expanded blood volume requires more iron to drive oxygen to the child and develop contraceptive organs. Counsel your primary care physician or enrolled dietitian nutritionist before taking an iron enhancement.

Small kids: Infants store sufficient iron for the initial half year of life. Following a half year, their iron necessities increase. Bosom milk and iron-sustained newborn child recipes can supply how much iron is not met by solids. Cow's milk is an unfortunate wellspring of iron. Whenever youngsters drink a lot of milk, they swarm out different food varieties and may create "milk sickness." The American Institute of Pediatrics suggests no cow's milk until the following year, so, all in all, it ought to be restricted to something like 4 cups each day.

Young adult Young ladies: Their frequently conflicting or confined eating fewer carbs — joined with fast development — put juvenile young ladies in danger.

Ladies of Childbearing Age: Ladies with unnecessarily weighty feminine periods might foster a lack of iron.

How to Prevent Iron Deficiency.

Eat a reasonable, sound eating routine that incorporates great wellsprings of lack of iron to forestall any. Join veggie lover wellsprings of iron with L-ascorbic acid in a similar dinner. For instance: a ringer pepper-bean salad, spinach with a lemon squeeze, or braced oat and berries.

If treatment for lack of iron is required, a medical care supplier will survey iron status and decide the specific type of therapy — which might remember changes in diet or taking enhancements.

Chapter.14

Iron.

Iron is a mineral, and its principal design is to convey oxygen in the hemoglobin of red platelets all through the body so cells can deliver energy. Iron likewise helps eliminate carbon dioxide. At the point when the body's iron stores become so low that insufficient ordinary red platelets can be made to convey oxygen proficiently, a condition known as lack of iron sickness is created.

At the point when levels of iron are low, weariness, shortcomings, and trouble keeping up with internal heat levels frequently result. Different side effects might include:

- Fair skin and fingernails
- Unsteadiness
- Migraine
- Glossitis (excited tongue)

Although iron is generally accessible in food, certain individuals, similar to juvenile young ladies and ladies ages 19 to 50 years of age may not get the sum they need consistently. It is likewise a worry for small kids and ladies who are pregnant or equipped for becoming pregnant. If treatment for lack of iron is required, a medical services supplier will evaluate the iron status and decide the specific type of therapy — which might remember changes in diet or potentially taking enhancements.

Infants need iron for mental health and development. They store sufficient iron for the initial four to a half years of life. An enhancement might be suggested by a pediatrician for a child that is untimely or a low-birth-weight and breastfed. Following a half year, their requirement for iron increments, so the presentation of strong food varieties when the child is formatively prepared can assist with giving wellsprings of iron. Most newborn child recipes are strengthened with iron.

How much iron do you want? While your body is truly adept at adjusting to lower or more significant levels by retaining pretty much iron depending on the situation, the prescribed levels are set to address the issues of the larger part of the populace. Here are the ongoing Suggested Dietary Remittances (RDAs) for iron:

- Orientation/Age Iron RDA
- Kids 1-3 7 mg
- Kids 4-8 10 mg
- Kids 9-13 8 mg
- Guys/14-18 11 mg
- Females/14-18 15 mg
- Guys/19+ 8 mg
- Females/19-50 18 mg
- Females/51+ 8 mg

Iron in food exists in two sorts, heme, and non-heme. Creature food sources, for example, meat, fish, and poultry give the two sorts and are better consumed by the body. Non-heme iron is tracked down in plant food varieties, for example, spinach and beans, grains that are improved, similar to rice and bread, and some strengthened breakfast cereals. To expand the retention of iron from plant sources, it's prescribed to eat them with meat, fish, or poultry or a decent wellspring of L-ascorbic acid, for example, citrus natural products, kiwi, strawberries, or ringer peppers. An effective method for further developing your iron admission is by eating a reasonable, sound eating regimen that incorporates different food sources.

Give Your Teens Iron a Boost.

What's the supplement most ailing in your adolescent's eating routine? While you could figure calcium, it very well may be iron.

- During adolescence (ages 9 to 13) both young men and young ladies need around 8 milligrams of iron every day. As teenagers develop, their bulk increments and blood volume grows, expanding their requirement for iron, so the proposal leaps to 15 milligrams of iron every day for young ladies ages 14 to 18, and 11 milligrams day to day for young men ages 14 to 18.

Notwithstanding the wealth of iron in the US food supply through regular, advanced, and sustained food sources, teenagers might be devouring less of this mineral than their creating bodies require. Young adult young ladies, particularly, will generally have lower admissions of food varieties that give iron. Kids and young people from food-shaky families are at a more serious gamble of not getting sufficient iron than their companions who have simpler admittance to food. Young ladies are additionally at increased hazard of lack of iron because of iron misfortune during the monthly cycle. Assuming adolescents are following calorie-prohibitive eating regimens to lose or oversee weight, that might influence iron admission, veggie lovers or vegetarian teenagers may likewise be in danger of not getting sufficient iron.

What does Iron do in the Body?

Iron assumes a huge part in numerous different capabilities since it assists the blood with conveying oxygen to the lungs, muscles, and all pieces of our bodies. Account of this job, additionally engaged with cerebrum capability and helps keep our safe framework solid.

A lack of iron may not give any indications or side effects or it might bring about a few, so, significantly, your kid's pediatrician assesses them. One normal sign is exhaustion. Different side effects might incorporate windedness; continuous colds and contaminations; unfortunate fixation; fair skin; discombobulation; unpredictable pulse; cerebral pains; and slender, fragile, and inward molded nails. Inadequate high schooler competitors might have dull instructional meetings and experience weariness during exercises.

The most effective method to Get More Iron.

Iron comes from different food sources: meat, poultry, and fish, as well as beans, nuts, improved grain items, and verdant green vegetables.

Creature wellsprings of iron (which contain heme iron) are all the more effectively consumed by the body, while plant sources (non-heme iron) ought to be eaten with an L-ascorbic acid source to assist with expanding its retention. For instance, serve iron-strengthened cereals with strawberries, and cook beans with tomatoes in a stew. Preparing food in a cast iron dish likewise can increment iron substance.

You can likewise check the Nourishment Realities Name for how much iron a food gives in light of the serving size that is recorded. The Percent Day to Day Worth (%DV) is a speedy method for distinguishing great sources. Search for a higher %DV of iron while contrasting food varieties, on the off chance that more iron is required.

A food source and refreshments might make the body ingest less iron when eaten near one another. An enlisted dietitian nutritionist can foster an eating plan that is ideal for your youngster and incorporates great wellsprings of iron with feasts and bites.

Taking an iron enhancement to address a lack of iron ought to be done exclusively under a doctor's oversight and checked with follow-up blood tests since high doses of iron from enhancements can be destructive, particularly for small kids.

Chapter.15

Water.

From greasing up joints to supporting processing, water is fundamental for the majority of physical processes. Figure out the amount you want to keep up with appropriate hydration.

How Much Water Do You Want?

With regards to how much water to drink every day, the vast majority recount the 8 x 8 rule. However, do you truly have to drink eight 8-ounce glasses, or 64 ounces, of water consistently?

Water is Vital for Life

Around 60% of your body is made of water. It assumes a part in keeping all of your body frameworks functioning admirably. Remaining very much hydrated can assist with lessening your gamble of creating kidney stones, urinary lot contaminations, and obstruction.

You lose water for the day with typical body processes, like making pee, having solid discharges, and perspiring. Extremely dynamic people can lose more water through sweat, as the body attempts to chill itself off. The equivalent is valid at higher elevations and when you are out in outrageous temperatures. Besides, ailments, for example, fever and looseness of the bowels bring about extra water misfortune.

The Risks of Dehydration and Overhydration.

Assuming that you lose more water than you take in, your body can become dried out. Drying out can unleash devastation on your body, causing migraines, dazedness, or absorption issues. A gentle lack of hydration might influence your state of mind, memory, or how well you're ready to deal with data. These side effects frequently disappear once your body gets rehydrated. Clinical consideration is frequently required with extreme parchedness since it can prompt more difficult issues like disarray, kidney disappointment, heart issues, and conceivably demise.

It is additionally conceivable to become overhydrated. Albeit this isn't as normal, competitors and people with specific ailments might be at a higher gamble for overhydration. Side effects of serious overhydration are frequently like lack of hydration and may likewise require clinical consideration. For instance, disarray and seizures can happen. People partaking in a significant length of active work, like long-distance races, frequently need to supplant both water and sodium misfortunes. On these occasions, a hydration plan is normally followed, and refreshments, for example, sports beverages might be suggested.

Liquid Necessities Differ.

Many elements influence how much water you want, including your age, sex, movement level, and by and large well-being. More water is required by people during pregnancy and keeping in mind breastfeeding. People with specific ailments, like congestive cardiovascular breakdown or renal infection, additionally have different liquid requirements. The equivalent is valid for those with serious diseases or runs.

Satisfactory admission levels for water are not entirely settled for commonly solid individuals and depend on age and sex.

For ladies, how much all out water is around 11.5 cups each day, and for men around 15.5 cups. These appraisals, be that as it may, incorporate liquids polished off from the two food sources and drinks, including water. You commonly get around 20% of the water you want from the food you eat. Considering that ladies need around nine cups of liquid each day and men around 13 cups to assist with renewing how much water that is lost.

Variety Check.

A fast and simple method for checking if you are getting sufficient water, in general, is to take a look at the shade of your pee. If you are sufficiently consuming, the pee variety will be a light yellow tone. On the off chance that it is a dim yellow or golden variety, you might have to expand the sum you consume.

Wellsprings of Water.

It's critical to supplant those water misfortunes to remain healthy. You can do this by partaking in different drinks, as well as eating food sources that have a high water content, like products of the soil. For drinks, centers around unsweetened refreshments, similar to water, to restrict calories from added sugars.

Ways Of expanding Water.

- Pay attention to your body: On the off chance that you are parched, hydrate. This is particularly significant assuming you are dynamic or live in exceptionally sweltering environments.
- Choose water: Rather than pop or caffeinated drinks, go with a fine specimen.
- Hydrate over the day: Drink water with dinners, as well as between feasts.
- Convey a refillable water bottle: Keep water helpful, so it's there when you need to go after a beverage.
- Add a flavor enhancer: For assortment, get some new lemon or lime juice into your water, throw in two or three cucumber cuts, or add a couple of new basil leaves.
-

Food sources That Are High in Water.

Choices with a 90-100 percent water content, include:

- Hydrates, shining water, and without fat milk.
- Natural products, particularly melon, strawberries, and watermelon.
- Vegetables like lettuce, cabbage, celery, spinach, and cooked squash.
-

Choices with a 70-89% water content, include:
- Organic products incorporate bananas, grapes, oranges, pears, and pineapples.
- Vegetables like carrots, cooked broccoli, and avocados.
- Dairy items like yogurt, curds, and ricotta cheddar.

At the point when Infants Need Additional Liquids.

Infants need no additional water. Bosom milk or baby recipes by and large will supply sufficient liquid to address their issues.

Assuming that your kid is debilitated with gentle loose bowels or heaving, continue breastfeeding assuming that you are nursing. Breastfeeding forestalls the runs, and your child might recuperate faster. Assuming you are utilizing equations, make it original capacity except if your medical services supplier offers you different guidance.

Contact your child's medical services supplier right away if:

- Your child is an infant (under 90 days old) and has looseness of the bowels.
- You see signs that your kid might be dried out, like dry lips, mouth, and tongue; no tears

while crying; no wet diaper for 3 hours; or quicker than a common heartbeat.

- Fever and looseness of the bowels or regurgitating go on for over 24 hours.

Check with your child's medical care supplier about supplanting liquids assuming your child is wiped out. The runs and heaving might prompt a lack of hydration — and make your child very wiped out — if liquids aren't supplanted. But instead of water, a game drink, or squeeze (which can exacerbate loose bowels), your PCP or pediatric medical caretaker might suggest an oral rehydration arrangement. These items are made explicitly for babies and kids. Other than liquid, the arrangement contains modest quantities of glucose (a type of sugar) and minerals (sodium, chloride, and potassium) called electrolytes. Electrolytes assist with keeping up with liquid equilibrium in your child's body cells. These minerals are lost with loose bowels or spewing. An oral rehydration arrangement won't stop the loose bowels or spewing, yet it forestalls the lack of hydration.

Before taking care of your baby or kid with an oral rehydration arrangement, counsel your youngster's medical services supplier. You actually must check with them as opposed to attempting to oversee swapping liquids for your child all alone, because other than the gamble of parchedness, loose bowels, and heaving might flag a sickness that requires clinical consideration. Staying away from lack of hydration is significant, yet that by itself doesn't tackle the fundamental issue.

Then again, the runs in children typically don't keep going long. Most frequently, it is brought about by an infection and disappears all alone, or is a transitory reaction to an adjustment of the child's (or a breastfeeding mother's) diet.

Water, How Much Do Kids Need?.

Water is one of the body's most fundamental supplements. Individuals might endure half a month with no food, however, they couldn't live more than a couple of days without water. That is because water is the foundation for all body capabilities. It's the most bountiful substance in the body, averaging around 50 to 70 percent of body weight. It assists keep with bodying temperature steady, transports supplements and oxygen to all cells, and diverts byproducts. Water keeps up with blood volume, and it greases up joints and body tissues like those in the mouth, eyes, and nose.

How Much Water Do Children Need?

The everyday measure of water that a kid needs relies upon variables like age, weight, and sex. Air temperature, dampness, action level, and an individual's general well-being influence day-to-day water necessities, as well. The graph underneath can assist you with distinguishing the number of cups of water your kid or adolescent requires every day. These proposals are set for commonly solid children living in mild environments; accordingly, they probably won't be precise for your youngster or adolescent.

How much water your kid or youngster needs every day is somewhat higher than the proposals in the outline. That is because how much all-out water an individual necessitates day to day incorporates water from all sources: drinking water, refreshments like milk, as well as food. Products of the soil have a lot higher water content than other strong food sources. This high water content assists keep the calorie evening out of products of the soil low while their supplement level remaining parts high — one more

128

smart justification behind children eating more from these nutrition types.

Chapter.16

Hydrate Right.

Appropriate hydration is one of the main parts of sound actual work. Drinking the perfect proportion of liquids previously, during, and after actual work is fundamental to giving your body the liquids it requires to appropriately perform. Sports dietitians help competitors by creating individualized hydration designs that improve execution in preparation and contest while limiting dangers for drying out, overhydration, and intensity ailment and injury.

Hydration Goal.

The general objective is to limit parchedness without over-drinking. Satisfactory hydration changes among people. Reasonable ways of observing hydration are:

- Pee tone. The shade of the main morning's pee void after arousing is a general mark of hydration status. Straw or lemonade-hued pee is an indication of suitable hydration. Dim-shaded pee, the shade of squeezed apple, shows parchedness. Splendid pee frequently is created not long after consuming nutrient enhancements.

- Sweet misfortune. Change in body weight when exercise is utilized to assess sweat misfortune. Since a competitor's perspiration misfortune during exercise is a sign of hydration status, competitors are encouraged to follow tweaked liquid substitution designs that consider thirst, pee tone, liquid admission, sweat misfortune, and body weight changes that happen during exercise.

Minimize Dehydration.

Parchedness can happen in basically every active work situation. It doesn't need to be hot. You don't have noticeable sweat. You can get dried out in the water, at a pool or lake, or skiing at a colder time of year.

Parchedness results when competitors neglect to supplant liquid lost by perspiring satisfactorily. Since parchedness that surpasses 2% body weight reduction hurts practice execution, competitors are encouraged to start practicing very much hydrated, limit drying out during exercise, and supplant liquid misfortunes after a workout.

Be ready for conditions that increment your liquid misfortune through sweat.

- Air Temperature: The higher the temperature, the more noteworthy your perspiration misfortunes.
- Power: The harder you figure out, the more you sweat.
- Body Size and Orientation: Bigger individuals sweat more. Men by and large perspiration more than ladies.
- Length: The more extended the exercise, the more liquid misfortune.
- Wellness: Thoroughly prepared competitors sweat more than less fit individuals. Why? Competitors cool their bodies through sweat more proficient than the vast majority because their bodies are utilized to the additional pressure. Consequently, liquid requirements are higher for exceptionally prepared competitors than for less fit people.

Recollecting swimmers' sweat, as well. Like any athletic movement, when you swim, your internal heat level ascents, and your body sweat to hold back from overheating. You may not see since you are in the water, however, you can become dried out. Swimmers, from serious competitors to families sprinkling around, need to drink liquids previously, during, and in the wake of swimming, regardless of whether they feel parched.

Cautioning Signs.

Know the indications of parchedness. Early signs are:

- Thirst
- Flushed skin
- Untimely weariness
- Expanded internal heat level
- Quicker breathing and heartbeat rate
- Expanded impression of exertion
- Diminished practice limit

Later signs include:

- Wooziness
- Expanded shortcoming
- Worked breathing with workout

Fluid Replacement.

Supplant liquids during activity to advance satisfactory hydration. Hydrate instead of pouring it over your head. Drinking is the best way to rehydrate and cool your body from the back to the front. Sports drinks are more fitting than water for competitors participating in moderate-to-extreme focus practice that endures an hour or longer. Rehydrate after practice by drinking sufficient liquid to supplant liquid misfortunes during exercise.

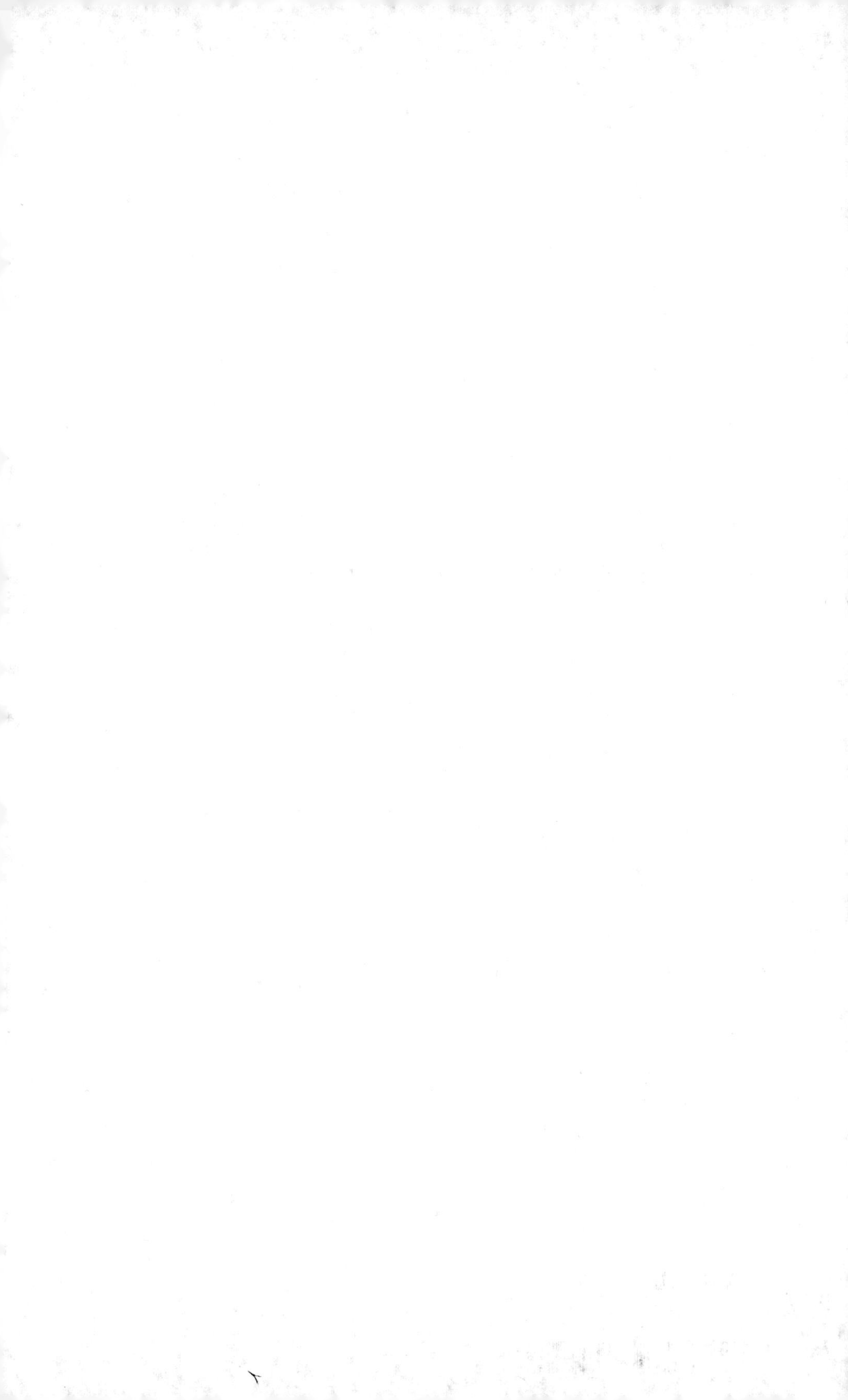